Prostate cancer: Prevention, treatment and management

Table of contents

Introduction

Prostate cancer is a common and often deadly disease that affects millions of men worldwide. It can be a difficult and scary topic to discuss, but it's one that needs to be addressed. In "Prostate Cancer: Prevention, Treatment, and Management," the author delve into the many facets of this complex disease. From the latest medical advances in diagnosis and treatment to tips on prevention and management. This comprehensive guide is a must-read for anyone affected by prostate cancer. Whether you're a patient, caregiver, or simply someone interested in learning more about this important topic, this book offers valuable insights and practical advice to help you navigate the challenges of prostate cancer with confidence and courage. So come along on this journey of discovery and learn how to take control of your prostate health today!

Helpful Quotes on Prostate Cancer

"Prostate cancer is not a death sentence. There are many ways to fight it and win." - Dr. Drew Pinsky

"Early detection is key when it comes to prostate cancer. Don't wait until it's too late." - Arnold Palmer

"Prostate cancer can be a wake-up call to make important changes in your life. Use it as an opportunity to prioritize your health and well-being." - Dr. David Samadi

"The most important thing a man can do to reduce his risk of prostate cancer is to take care of his overall health." - Dr. Mark Moyad

"Prostate cancer is a journey, not a destination. It's important to stay positive and keep fighting." - Dan Haggerty

"Don't be afraid to talk about prostate cancer. The more we talk about it, the more we can do to prevent it and find a cure." - Harry Belafonte

"Prostate cancer doesn't discriminate. It can affect men of all ages, races, and backgrounds." - Dr. William J. Catalona

"Education is the best weapon against prostate cancer. Know your risk factors, get screened regularly, and make informed decisions about your health." - Dr. Mehmet Oz

"The best way to beat prostate cancer is to catch it early and take action. Don't wait until it's too late." - Joe Torre

Chapter One

Prostate cancer survival

Survival from prostate cancer depends on various factors, such as the stage of cancer, age, overall health, and response to treatment. Here are some ways to increase your chances of surviving prostate cancer:

- Early detection: Regular prostate cancer screening is essential, especially for men at higher risk of developing prostate cancer. Prostate cancer is often asymptomatic in its early stages, and screening can help detect cancer before it spreads.

- Treatment options: Treatment options for prostate cancer include surgery, radiation therapy, hormone therapy, chemotherapy, and immunotherapy. Your doctor will determine the best treatment option based on the stage of cancer, your overall health, and other factors.

- Healthy lifestyle: A healthy lifestyle can help reduce the risk of prostate cancer and improve survival chances. This includes eating a balanced diet, exercising regularly, maintaining a healthy weight, and avoiding tobacco and excessive alcohol consumption.

- Support system: A strong support system, including family, friends, and healthcare providers, can help you manage the physical and emotional effects of prostate cancer and treatment.

It's important to remember that prostate cancer is treatable, and survival rates are generally good, especially when the cancer is detected early. Talk to your doctor about the best ways to manage and survive prostate cancer.

Surviving prostate cancer through food and diet.

Prostate cancer is a serious disease that affects the prostate gland in men. While a healthy diet cannot cure prostate cancer, it can help improve a patient's overall health and quality of life. Below are some ways to survive prostate cancer through food and diet.

- Eat a diet rich in fruits and vegetables: Studies have shown that a diet high in fruits and vegetables can help lower the risk of prostate cancer. Aim for at least five servings of fruits and vegetables per day.

- Include whole grains in your diet: Whole grains such as brown rice, quinoa, and whole wheat bread are rich in fiber and can help keep you feeling full and satisfied. They also contain important nutrients that can help support your immune system.

- Choose lean protein sources: Opt for lean protein sources such as chicken, fish, and tofu instead of red meat. Red meat is high in saturated fat, which can increase the risk of prostate cancer.

- Eat foods rich in omega-3 fatty acids: Omega-3 fatty acids are important for heart health and may also help lower the risk of prostate cancer. Foods rich in omega-3s include fatty fish like salmon, flaxseeds, and chia seeds.

- Limit your intake of processed foods: Processed foods are often high in salt, sugar, and unhealthy fats. These foods can contribute to inflammation in the body, which may increase the risk of prostate cancer, so they should be vehemently avoided.

- Stay hydrated: Drinking plenty of water is important for overall health, and it can also help prevent constipation, a common side effect of cancer treatment. It is very important to stay hydrated to survive prostate cancer.

- Consult with a registered dietitian: A registered dietitian can help you create a personalized nutrition plan based on your individual needs and preferences. They can also help you manage side effects of cancer treatment, such as nausea and weight loss.

It's important to remember that diet alone cannot cure prostate cancer, but eating a healthy diet can help support overall health and well-being during cancer treatment. Always consult with your healthcare provider before making any changes to your diet or lifestyle.

Chapter Two

Some excellent prostate cancer preventive advice.

- Get regular check-ups: It's important to get regular check-ups and screenings for prostate cancer, especially if you're over the age of 50 or have a family history of prostate cancer.

- Maintain a healthy diet: A diet high in fruits, vegetables, and whole grains and low in saturated and trans fats can reduce your risk of prostate cancer.

- Exercise regularly: Regular physical activity can help reduce your risk of prostate cancer. Aim for at least 30 minutes of moderate exercise most days of the week.

- Maintain a healthy weight: Being overweight or obese can increase your risk of prostate cancer, so it's important to maintain a healthy weight.

- Quit smoking: Smoking has been linked to an increased risk of prostate cancer, so quitting smoking can help reduce your risk.

- Limit alcohol consumption: Drinking alcohol in moderation is generally safe, but heavy drinking can increase your risk of prostate cancer.

- Consider prostate cancer screening: Talk to your doctor about whether prostate cancer screening is appropriate for you based on your age, family history, and other factors.

Remember, early detection is key to successful treatment of prostate cancer.

prostate cancer prevention through food and diet

Prostate cancer is a type of cancer that affects the prostate gland, which is located below the bladder in men. While there is no guaranteed way to prevent prostate cancer, research suggests that a healthy diet can help reduce the risk of developing the disease. Below are some dietary recommendations for prostate cancer prevention.

- Eat a variety of fruits and vegetables: Fruits and vegetables are packed with vitamins, minerals, and antioxidants, which can help protect against cancer. Aim to include a variety of different colored fruits and vegetables in your diet, such as berries, leafy greens, carrots, and tomatoes.

- Choose whole grains: Whole grains like brown rice, whole-wheat bread, and quinoa are a good source of fiber and other nutrients that can help reduce the risk of prostate cancer.

- Include healthy fats: Omega-3 fatty acids, found in fatty fish like salmon and sardines, as well as nuts and seeds like flaxseed and chia seeds, have been shown to reduce inflammation and may help lower the risk of prostate cancer.

- Limit red meat and processed meats: High consumption of red meat and processed meats like bacon and sausage have been linked to an increased risk of prostate cancer. Try to limit your intake of these foods and opt for leaner protein sources like chicken, fish, and legumes instead.

- Reduce dairy consumption: While dairy products are a good source of calcium, high intake of dairy products has been linked to an increased risk of prostate cancer. Consider reducing your intake of dairy or choosing low-fat or non-dairy alternatives like almond or soy milk.

- Drink green tea: Green tea is a rich source of antioxidants called catechins, which have been shown to have anti-cancer properties. Aim to drink 2-3 cups of green tea per day.

- Maintain a healthy weight: Obesity and being overweight have been linked to an increased risk of prostate cancer. Aim to maintain a healthy weight through a balanced diet and regular exercise.

Without mincing matters, a healthy diet rich in fruits and vegetables, whole grains, and healthy fats, and low in red meat, processed meats, and dairy products, may help reduce the risk of prostate cancer.

Chapter Three

Strategies for Managing Prostate Cancer.

Prostate cancer is a type of cancer that develops in the prostate gland, which is a walnut-sized gland that produces semen in men. Treatment strategies for prostate cancer depend on various factors such as the stage of cancer, the age and overall health of the patient, and the patient's preferences. Explained below are some common management strategies for prostate cancer.

- Active Surveillance: This approach involves closely monitoring the patient's prostate cancer with regular PSA (prostate-specific antigen) tests, digital rectal exams, and imaging tests. Treatment is only initiated if there are any signs of disease progression.

- Surgery: Surgical removal of the prostate gland, known as prostatectomy, is an option for patients with localized prostate cancer. The surgeon may use open surgery or minimally invasive techniques such as laparoscopic or robotic-assisted surgery.

- Radiation Therapy: This involves using high-energy X-rays or other types of radiation to destroy cancer cells. Radiation therapy can be given externally or internally.

- Hormone Therapy: Hormone therapy involves blocking the production or action of testosterone, which can help slow the growth of prostate cancer.

- Chemotherapy: Chemotherapy involves using drugs to kill cancer cells. It is usually reserved for advanced prostate cancer cases that have spread to other parts of the body.

- Immunotherapy: Immunotherapy involves using drugs to boost the body's immune system to fight cancer cells.

- Bone-Directed Therapy: This approach is used to treat prostate cancer that has spread to the bones. It includes medications that strengthen bones and medications that help relieve pain.

It is important to note that the treatment options and management strategies for prostate cancer vary for each patient. A multidisciplinary team consisting of urologists, radiation oncologists, medical oncologists, and other healthcare professionals can work together to develop an individualized treatment plan for each patient.

Prostate Cancer Survivorship

Prostate cancer is a type of cancer that develops in the prostate, a gland in the male reproductive system. It is the second most common type of cancer in men worldwide, and the risk increases with age.

Surviving prostate cancer can be a challenging experience, as it involves physical, emotional, and psychological changes. The treatment for prostate cancer varies depending on the stage and severity of the cancer, and may include surgery, radiation therapy, hormone therapy, chemotherapy, or a combination of these treatments.

Many men who survive prostate cancer experience side effects from treatment, including urinary incontinence, erectile dysfunction, fatigue, and changes in bowel habits. These side effects can have a significant impact on a man's quality of life and may require ongoing support and treatment.

However, there are many resources available to support prostate cancer survivors, including support groups, counseling, and rehabilitation programs. These programs can help men manage their physical and emotional health and navigate the challenges of survivorship.

If you or a loved one is a prostate survivor, it's essential to work with your healthcare team to develop a plan for ongoing care and support. This may include regular check-ups, monitoring for recurrence, and on going management of any treatment-related side effects.

There are also many advocacy organizations dedicated to supporting prostate cancer survivors, including the Prostate Cancer Foundation, the American Cancer Society, and the National Comprehensive Cancer Network. These organizations can provide information, resources, and support for men and their families affected by prostate cancer.

Remember, every survivor's experience is unique, and it's essential to prioritize self-care and seek support as needed throughout the survivorship journey.

Chapter four

Prostate Cancer Prevention, treatment and management: Medicinal herbs/plant

Medicinal herbs that could help to prevent prostate cancer.

There are several medicinal herbs that have been studied for their potential to prevent prostate cancer. Here are a few.

- Saw Palmetto: Saw Palmetto is a plant that grows in North America and has been used traditionally to treat prostate problems. It is thought to work by inhibiting the enzyme that converts testosterone to dihydrotestosterone (DHT), which is a hormone that can stimulate the growth of prostate cells.

- Green Tea: Green tea contains compounds called catechins that have been shown to have anti-cancer properties. One study found that men who drank green tea regularly had a lower risk of developing prostate cancer than those who didn't.

- Turmeric: Turmeric is a spice that contains a compound called curcumin, which has anti-inflammatory properties. Inflammation has been linked to the development of prostate cancer, so turmeric may help to prevent it.

- Garlic: Garlic contains a compound called allicin, which has been shown to have anti-cancer properties. One study found that men who ate garlic regularly had a lower risk of developing prostate cancer than those who didn't.

- Pomegranate: Pomegranate contains compounds called ellagitannins, which have been shown to have anti-cancer properties. One study found that men who drank pomegranate juice regularly had slower prostate cancer growth than those who didn't.

- Onion: Onions has anti-cancer properties and eating it regularly and preferably raw, will help your entire body system to fight cancerous growth and tumors.

It's important to note that while these herbs may have some potential benefits for preventing prostate cancer, more research is needed to fully understand their effects and to determine safe and effective doses. It's also important to consult with a healthcare provider before starting any new herbal supplement.

These medicinal herbs should be taken regularly and on a daily basis to help prevent, treat and overcome prostate cancer problems.

Prostate cancer diet.

There is no specific diet that can cure or prevent prostate cancer, but research suggests that a healthy diet may help reduce the risk of developing prostate cancer and may also aid in the treatment of the disease. Below are some dietary recommendations for prostate cancer.

- Eat a diet that is rich in fruits and vegetables: Eating a variety of colorful fruits and vegetables can provide antioxidants, fiber, and other important nutrients that can help lower the risk of prostate cancer. Aim for at least 5 servings of fruits and vegetables each day.

- Choose whole grains: Whole-grain breads, cereals, pasta, and rice are rich in fiber and other important nutrients that may help reduce the risk of prostate cancer. Try to choose whole grains over refined grains whenever possible.

- Include healthy fats in your diet: Healthy fats such as omega-3 fatty acids, found in fatty fish like salmon, can help reduce inflammation in the body. Other sources of healthy fats include nuts, seeds, and olive oil.

- Limit intake of red and processed meats: Red and processed meats have been linked to an increased risk of prostate cancer, so it is recommended to limit their intake.

- Drink green tea: Green tea contains antioxidants that may help prevent the growth of prostate cancer cells. Try drinking 2-3 cups of green tea each day.

- Pomegranate juice: Making pomegranate juice a daily routine or taking pomegranate juice extract can significantly aid in the treatment of prostate cancer. So incorporate it into your everyday diet.

It is important to note that dietary changes alone cannot cure or prevent prostate cancer, but they can be a helpful addition to other treatments recommended by your doctor. Consult with a healthcare professional for personalized dietary recommendations.